Healthy Plant Based Diet Cookbook

Creative & Healthy Plant Based Meals

Jason Noel

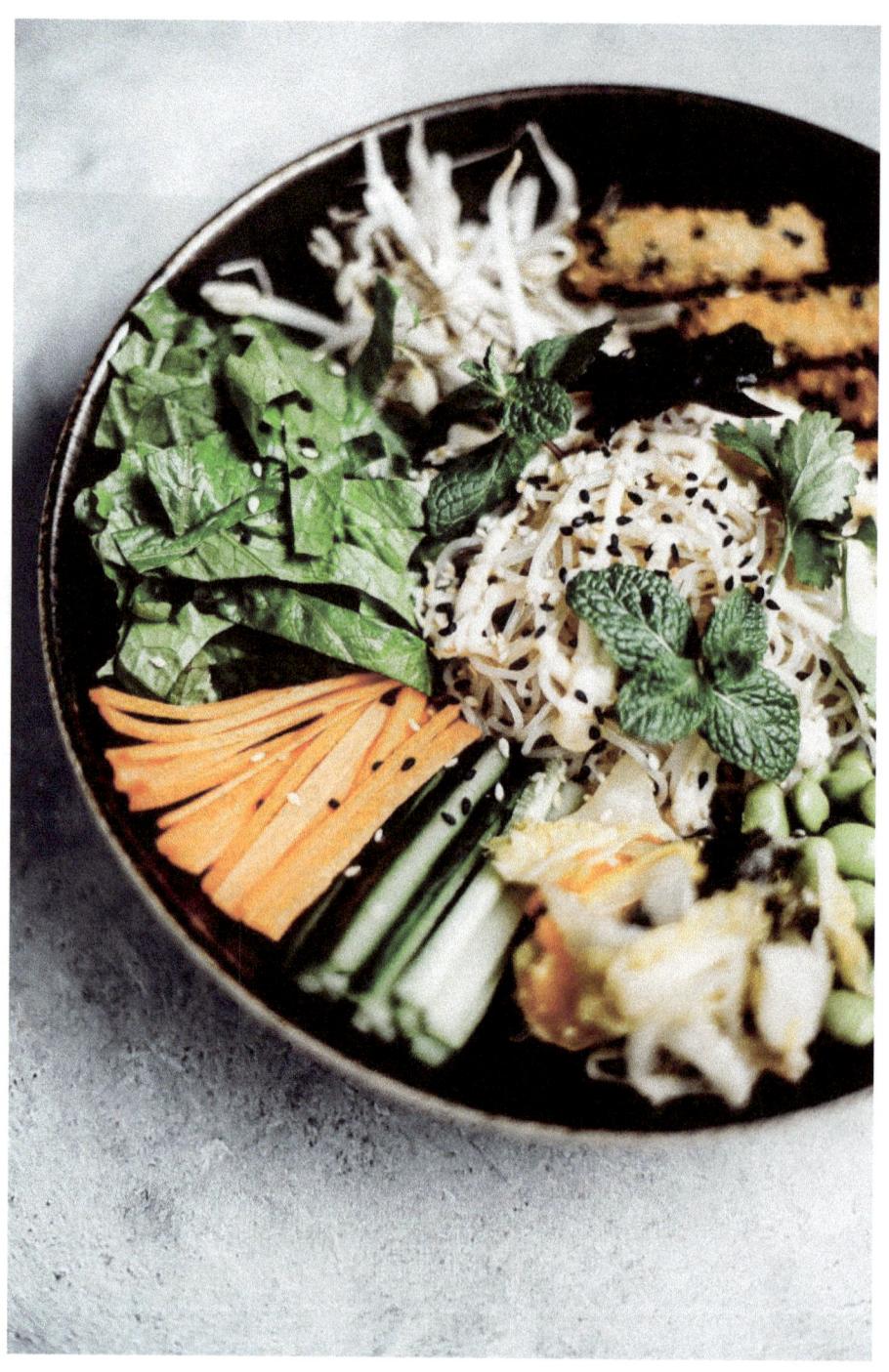

© Copyright 2021 - All rights reserved.

The content contained within this book may not be reproduced, duplicated or transmitted without direct written permission from the author or the publisher.
Under no circumstances will any blame or legal responsibility be held against the publisher, or author, for any damages, reparation, or monetary loss due to the information contained within this book. Either directly or indirectly.

Legal Notice:
This book is copyright protected. This book is only for personal use. You cannot amend, distribute, sell, use, quote or paraphrase any part, or the content within this book, without the consent of the author or publisher.

Disclaimer Notice:
Please note the information contained within this document is for educational and entertainment purposes only. All effort has been executed to present accurate, up to date, and reliable, complete information. No warranties of any kind are declared or implied. Readers acknowledge that the author is not engaging in the rendering of legal, financial, medical or professional advice. The content within this book has been derived from various sources. Please consult a licensed professional before attempting any techniques outlined in this book.
By reading this document, the reader agrees that under no circumstances is the author responsible for any losses, direct or indirect, which are incurred as a result of the use of information contained within this document, including, but not limited to, — errors, omissions, or inaccuracies.

Table of Contents

LENTIL, RICE AND VEGETABLE BAKE	7
TANGY TOFU MEATLOAF	9
VEGAN BACON-WRAPPED TOFU WITH BUTTERED SPINACH	11
SEITAN ZOODLE BOWL	13
TOFU PARSNIP BAKE	15
SQUASH TEMPEH LASAGNA	17
BOK CHOY TOFU SKILLET	19
FENNEL AND CHICKPEAS PROVENÇAL	21
TOFU FAJITA BOWL	23
INDIAN STYLE TEMPEH BAKE	25
TOFU- SEITAN CASSEROLE	27
GINGER LIME TEMPEH	29
TOFU MOZZARELLA	31
SEITAN MEATZA WITH KALE	33
BROCCOLI TEMPEH	35
AVOCADO SEITAN	37
JAMAICAN JERK TEMPEH	39
CURRIED TOFU MEATBALLS	41
SPICY MUSHROOM COLLARD WRAPS	43
PESTO TOFU ZOODLES	45
CHEESY MUSHROOM PIE	47

- TOFU SCALLOPINI WITH LEMON 50
- TOFU CHOPS WITH GREEN BEANS AND AVOCADO SAUTÉ 53
- MUSHROOM IN TORTILLAS 55
- HAZELNUTS AND CHEESE STUFFED ZUCCHINIS 58
- TEMPEH STUFFED MUSHROOMS 60
- MUSHROOM AND VEGAN BACON LETTUCE WRAPS 62
- MUSHROOM IN THAI CURRY SAUCE 64
- BAKED CAMEMBERT CHEESE WITH SEITAN AND PECANS 66
- CHEESY TEMPEH BURRITO BOWL 68
- TOFU CASSEROLE WITH COTTAGE CHEESE 70
- EGG ROLL AND TOFU BOWL 72
- PIZZA ALLA PUTTANESCA 74
- SEITAN FAJITAS 77
- ZESTY STUFFED BELL PEPPERS 79
- MOROCCAN STUFFED PEPPERS 81
- TEMPEH CHOPS WITH CARAMELIZED ONIONS AND BRIE CHEESE 85
- BROWN RICE STIR FRY WITH VEGETABLES 87
- GRILLED VEGGIE SKEWERS 89
- EGGPLANT TERIYAKI BOWLS 91
- QUINOA AND BLACK BEAN CHILLI 93
- BROCCOLI MAC AND CHEESE 96
- BUTTERNUT SQUASH LINGUINE WITH FRIED SAGE 98

PAELLA	100
SPICY THAI PEANUT SAUCE OVER ROASTED SWEET POTATOES AND RICE	103
CHICKPEA BIRYANI	106
CHINESE EGGPLANT	108
BLACK PEPPER TOFU WITH BOK CHOY	110

Lentil, Rice and Vegetable Bake

Preparation Time: 10 minutes | Cooking Time: 40 minutes | Servings: 6

Ingredients:

- 1/2 cup white rice, cooked
- 1 cup red lentils, cooked
- 1/3 cup chopped carrots
- 1 medium tomato, chopped
- 1 small onion, peeled, chopped
- 1/3 cup chopped zucchini
- 1/3 cup chopped celery
- 1 ½ teaspoon minced garlic
- ½ teaspoon ground black pepper
- 1 teaspoon dried basil
- 1 teaspoon ground cumin
- 1 teaspoon dried oregano
- ½ teaspoon salt

- 1 teaspoon olive oil

- 8 ounces tomato sauce

Directions:

- Take a skillet pan, place it over medium heat, add oil, and when hot, add onion and garlic and cook for 5 minutes.

- Then add remaining vegetables, season with salt, black pepper, and half of each cumin, oregano, and basil, and cook for 5 minutes until vegetables are tender.

- Take a casserole dish, place lentils and rice in it, top with vegetables, spread with tomato sauce and sprinkle with remaining cumin, oregano, and basil, and bake for 30 minutes until bubbly.

- Serve straight away.

Nutrition:

Calories: 187 Cal | Fat: 1.5 g | Carbs: 35.1 g | Protein: 9.7 g | Fiber: 8.1 g

Tangy Tofu Meatloaf

Preparation Time: 10 minutes | Cooking Time: 40 minutes | Servings: 6

Ingredients:

- 2 ½ lb ground tofu
- Salt and ground black pepper to taste
- 3 tbsp flaxseed meal
- 2 large eggs
- 2 tbsp olive oil
- 1 lemon, 1 tbsp juiced
- ¼ cup freshly chopped parsley
- ¼ cup freshly chopped oregano
- 4 garlic cloves, minced
- Lemon slices to garnish

Directions:

- Preheat the oven to 400 F and grease a loaf pan with cooking spray. Set aside.

- In a large bowl, combine the tofu, salt, black pepper, and flaxseed meal. Set aside.

- In a small bowl, whisk the eggs with the olive oil, lemon juice, parsley, oregano, and garlic. Pour the mixture onto the mix and combine well.

- Spoon the tofu mixture into the loaf pan and press to fit into the pan. Bake in the middle rack of the oven for 30 to 40 minutes.

- Remove the pan, tilt to drain the meat's liquid, and allow cooling for 5 minutes. • Slice, garnish with some lemon slices, and serve with braised green beans.

Nutrition:

Calories:238 | Total Fat:26.3g | Saturated Fat:14.9g | Total Carbs:1g | Dietary Fiber:0g | Sugar:0g | Protein:1g | Sodium:183mg

Vegan Bacon-Wrapped Tofu with Buttered Spinach

Preparation Time: 5 minutes | Cooking Time: 20 minutes | Servings: 4

Ingredients:

- For the bacon-wrapped tofu:
- 4 tofu
- 8 slices vegan bacon
- Salt and black pepper to taste
- 2 tbsp olive oil
- For the buttered spinach:
- 2 tbsp butter
- 1 lb spinach
- 4 garlic cloves
- Salt and ground black pepper to taste

Directions:

- For the bacon-wrapped tofu:

- Preheat the oven to 450 F.

- Wrap each tofu with two vegan bacon slices, season with salt and black pepper, and place on the baking sheet. Drizzle with the olive oil and bake in the oven for 15 minutes or until the vegan bacon browns and the tofu cooks within.

- For the buttered spinach:

- Meanwhile, melt the butter in a large skillet, add and sauté the spinach and garlic until the leaves wilt, 5 minutes. Season with salt and black pepper.

- Remove the tofu from the oven and serve with the buttered spinach.

Nutrition:

Calories:260 | Total Fat:24.7g | Saturated Fat:14.3g | Total Carbs:4g | Dietary Fiber:0g | Sugar:2g | Protein:6g | Sodium:215mg

Seitan Zoodle Bowl

Preparation Time: 15 minutes | Cooking Time: 13 minutes | Servings: 4

Ingredients:

- 5 garlic cloves, minced, divided
- ¼ tsp pureed onion
- Salt and ground black pepper to taste
- 2 ½ lb Seitan, cut into strips
- 2 tbsp avocado oil
- 3 large eggs, lightly beaten
- ¼ cup vegetable broth
- 2 tbsp coconut aminos
- 1 tbsp white vinegar
- ½ cup freshly chopped scallions
- 1 tsp red chili flakes
- 4 medium zucchinis, spiralized
- ½ cup toasted pine nuts, for topping

Directions:

- In a medium bowl, combine half of the pureed garlic, onion, salt, and black pepper. Add the seitan and mix well.

- Heat the avocado oil in a large, deep skillet over medium heat and add the seitan. Cook for 8 minutes. Transfer to a plate.

- Pour the eggs into the pan and scramble for 1 minute. Spoon the eggs to the side of the seitan and set aside.

- Reduce the heat to low and in a medium bowl, mix the vegetable broth, coconut aminos, vinegar, scallions, remaining garlic, and red chili flakes. Mix well and simmer for 3 minutes.

- Stir in the seitan, zucchini, and eggs. Cook for 1 minute and turn the heat off. Adjust the taste with salt and black pepper.

- Spoon the zucchini food into serving plates, top with the pine nuts and serve warm.

Nutrition:

Calories:687 | Total Fat:54.5g | Saturated Fat:27.4g | Total Carbs:9g |, Dietary Fiber:2g | Sugar:4g |, Protein:38g | Sodium:883mg

Tofu Parsnip Bake

Preparation Time: 5 minutes | Cooking Time: 44 minutes | Servings: 4

Ingredients:
- 6 vegan bacon slices, chopped
- 2 tbsp butter
- ½ lb parsnips, peeled and diced
- 2 tbsp olive oil
- 1 lb ground tofu
- Salt and ground black pepper to taste
- 2 tbsp butter
- 1 cup full- fat heavy cream
- 2 oz dairy-free cream cheese (vegan), softened
- 1 ¼ cups grated cheddar cheese
- ¼ cup chopped scallions

Directions:
- Preheat the oven to 300 F and lightly grease a baking dish with cooking spray. Set aside.

- Put the vegan bacon in a medium pot and fry on both sides until brown and crispy, 7 minutes. Spoon onto a plate and set aside.

- Melt the butter in a large skillet and sauté the parsnips until softened and lightly browned. Transfer to the baking sheet and set aside.

- Heat the olive oil in the same pan and cook the tofu (seasoned with salt and black pepper). Spoon onto a plate and set aside too.

- Add the butter, full-fat heavy cream, cashew cream, two-thirds of the cheddar cheese, salt, and black pepper to the pot. Melt the ingredients over medium heat with frequent stirring, 7 minutes.

- Spread the parsnips in the baking dish, top with the tofu, pour the full- fat heavy cream mixture over, and scatter the top with the vegan bacon and scallions.

- Sprinkle the remaining cheese on top, and bake in the oven until the cheese melts and is golden, 30 minutes.

- Remove the dish, spoon the food into serving plates, and serve immediately.

Nutrition:
Calories:534 | Total Fat:56g | Saturated Fat:34.6g | Total Carbs:4g | Dietary Fiber:1g | Sugar:1g | Protein:7g | Sodium:430mg

Squash Tempeh Lasagna

Preparation Time: 15 minutes | Cooking Time: 40 minutes | Servings: 4

Ingredients:
- 2 tbsp butter
- 1 ½ lb ground tempeh
- Salt and ground black pepper to taste
- 1 tsp garlic powder
- 1 tsp onion powder
- 2 tbsp coconut flour
- 1 ½ cup grated mozzarella cheese
- 1/3 cup parmesan cheese
- 2 cups crumbled cottage cheese
- 1 large egg, beaten into a bowl
- 2 cups unsweetened marinara sauce
- 1 tbsp dried Italian mixed herbs
- ¼ tsp red chili flakes
- 4 large yellow squash, sliced
- ¼ cup fresh basil leaves

Directions:
- Preheat the oven to 375 F and grease a baking dish with cooking spray. Set aside.

- Melt the butter in a large skillet over medium heat and cook the tempeh until brown, 10 minutes. Set aside to cool.

- In a medium bowl, mix the garlic powder, onion powder, coconut flour, salt, black pepper, mozzarella cheese, half of the parmesan cheese, cottage cheese, and egg. Set aside. • In another bowl, combine the marinara sauce, mixed herbs, and red chili flakes. Set aside.

- Make a single layer of the squash slices in the baking dish; spread a quarter of the egg mixture on top, a layer of the tempeh, then a quarter of the marinara sauce. Repeat the layering process in the same ingredient proportions and sprinkle the top with the remaining parmesan cheese.

- Bake in the oven until golden brown on top, 30 minutes.

- Remove the dish from the oven, allow cooling for 5 minutes, garnish with the basil leaves, slice, and serve.

Nutrition:
Calories:194 | Total Fat:17.4g | Saturated Fat:2.1g | Total Carbs:7g | Dietary Fiber:3g | Sugar:2g | Protein:7g | Sodium:72mg

Bok Choy Tofu Skillet

Preparation Time: 10 minutes | Cooking Time: 18 minutes | Servings: 4

Ingredients:

- 2 lb tofu, cut into 1-inch cubes

- Salt and ground black pepper to taste

- 4 vegan bacon slices, chopped

- 1 tbsp coconut oil

- 1 orange bell pepper, deseeded, cut into chunks

- 2 cups baby bok choy

- 2 tbsp freshly chopped oregano

- 2 garlic cloves, pressed

Directions:

- Season the tofu with salt and black pepper, and set aside.

- Heat a large skillet over medium heat and fry the vegan bacon until brown and crispy. Transfer to a plate.

- Melt the coconut oil in the skillet and cook the tofu until golden-brown and cooked through, 10 minutes. Remove onto the vegan bacon plate and set aside.

- Add the bell pepper and bok choy to the skillet and sauté until softened, 5 minutes. Stir in the vegan bacon, tofu, oregano, and garlic. Season with salt and black pepper and cook for 3 minutes or until the flavors incorporate. Turn the heat off.

- Plate the dish and serve with cauliflower rice.

Nutrition:

Calories:273 | Total Fat:18.7g | Saturated Fat:7.9g | Total Carbs:15g | Dietary Fiber:4g |, Sugar:8g | Protein:15g | Sodium:341mg

Fennel and Chickpeas Provençal

Preparation Time: 10 minutes | Cooking Time: 50 minutes | Servings: 4

Ingredients:

- 15 ounces cooked chickpeas
- 3 fennel bulbs, sliced
- 1 medium onion, peeled, sliced
- 15 ounces diced tomatoes
- 10 black olives, pitted, cured
- 10 Kalamata olives, pitted
- 1 ½ teaspoon minced garlic
- 1 teaspoon salt
- 1/8 teaspoon ground black pepper
- 1 teaspoon Herbes de Provence
- 1/2 teaspoon red pepper flakes
- 2 tablespoons olive oil
- 1/2 cup water

- 2 tablespoons chopped parsley

Directions:

- Take a saucepan, place it over medium-high heat, add oil, and when hot, add onion, fennel, and garlic and cook for 20 minutes until softened.

- Then add remaining ingredients except for olives and chickpeas, bring the mixture to boil, switch heat to medium-low level and simmer for 15 minutes.

- Then add remaining ingredients, cook for 10 minutes until hot, garnish stew with parsley and serve.

Nutrition:

Calories: 395 Cal | Fat: 13 g | Carbs: 56 g | Protein: 16 g | Fiber: 13 g

Tofu Fajita Bowl

Preparation Time: 5minutes | Cooking Time: 10minutes | Servings: 4

Ingredients:

- 2 tbsp olive oil
- 1½ lb tofu, cut into strips
- Salt and ground black pepper to taste
- 2 tbsp Tex-Mex seasoning
- 1 small iceberg lettuce, chopped
- 2 large tomatoes, deseeded and chopped
- 2 avocados, halved, pitted, and chopped
- 1 green bell pepper, deseeded and thinly sliced
- 1 yellow onion, thinly sliced
- 4 tbsp fresh cilantro leaves
- ½ cup shredded dairy-free parmesan cheese blend
- 1 cup plain unsweetened yogurt

Directions:

• Heat the olive oil in a medium skillet over medium heat, season the tofu with salt, black pepper, and Tex-Mex seasoning. Fry in the oil on both sides until golden and cooked, 5 to 10 minutes. Transfer to a plate.

• Divide the lettuce into 4 serving bowls, share the tofu on top, and add the tomatoes, avocados, bell pepper, onion, cilantro, and cheese.

• Top with dollops of plain yogurt and serve immediately with low carb tortillas.

Nutrition:

• Calories:263 | Total Fat:26.4g | Saturated Fat:8.8g | Total Carbs:4g | Dietary Fiber:1g | Sugar:3g | Protein:4g | Sodium:826mg

Indian Style Tempeh Bake

Preparation Time: 10minutes | Cooking Time: 26minutes | Servings: 4

Ingredients:

- 3 tbsp unsalted butter
- 6 tempeh, cut into 1-inch cubes
- Salt and ground black pepper to taste
- 2 ½ tbsp garam masala
- 1 cup baby spinach, tightly pressed
- 1¼ cups coconut cream
- 1 tbsp fresh cilantro, finely chopped

Directions:

- Preheat the oven to 350 F and grease a baking dish with cooking spray. Set aside.
- Heat the ghee in a medium skillet over medium heat, season the tempeh with salt and black

pepper, and cook in the oil on both sides until golden on the outside, 6 minutes.

• Mix in half of the garam masala and transfer the tempeh (with juices into the baking dish.

• Add the spinach, and spread the coconut cream on top. Bake in the oven for 20 minutes or until the cream is bubbly.

• Remove the dish, garnish with cilantro, and serve with cauliflower couscous.

Nutrition:

Calories:598 | Total Fat:56g | Saturated Fat:18.8g | Total Carbs12:g | Dietary Fiber:3g | Sugar:5g | Protein:15g | Sodium:762mg

Tofu- Seitan Casserole

Preparation Time: 10minutes | Cooking Time: 20minutes | Servings: 4

Ingredients:

- 1 tofu, shredded
- 7 oz seitan, chopped
- 8 oz dairy-free cream cheese (vegan
- 1 tbsp Dijon mustard
- 1 tbsp plain vinegar
- 10 oz shredded cheddar cheese
- Salt and ground black pepper to taste

Directions:

- Preheat the oven to 350 F and grease a baking dish with cooking spray. Set aside.
- Spread the tofu and seitan in the bottom of the dish.
- In a small bowl, mix the cashew cream, Dijon mustard, vinegar, and two-thirds of the

cheddar cheese. Spread the mixture on top of the tofu and seitan, season with salt and black pepper, and cover with the remaining cheese.

- Bake in the oven for 15 to 20 minutes or until the cheese melts and is golden brown.

- Remove the dish and serve with steamed collards.

Nutrition:

Calories475 | Total Fat:41.2g | Saturated Fat:12.3g | Total Carbs:6g | Dietary Fiber:3g | Sugar:2g | Protein:24g | Sodium:755mg

Ginger Lime Tempeh

Preparation Time: 10 minutes | Cooking Time: 40 minutes | Servings: 4

Ingredients:

- 5 kaffir lime leaves
- 1 tbsp cumin powder
- 1 tbsp ginger powder
- 1 cup plain unsweetened yogurt
- 2 lb tempeh
- Salt and ground black pepper to taste
- 1 tbsp olive oil
- 2 limes, juiced

Directions:

- In a large bowl, combine the kaffir lime leaves, cumin, ginger, and plain yogurt. Add the tempeh, season with salt, and black pepper, and mix to coat well. Cover the bowl with a plastic wrap and marinate in the refrigerator for 2 to 3 hours.

- Preheat the oven to 350 F and grease a baking sheet with cooking spray.

- Take out the tempeh and arrange it on the baking sheet. Drizzle with olive oil, lime juice, cover with aluminum foil, and slow-cook in the oven for 1 to 1 ½ hours or until the tempeh cooks within.

- Remove the aluminum foil, turn the broiler side of the oven on, and brown the top of the tempeh for 5 to 10 minutes.

- Take out the tempeh and serve warm with red cabbage slaw.

Nutrition:

Calories:285 | Total Fat:25.6g | Saturated Fat:13.6g |, Total Carbs:7g | Dietary Fiber:2g | Sugar:2g | Protein:11g |, Sodium:772mg

Tofu Mozzarella

Preparation Time: 10minutes | Cooking Time: 35minutes | Servings: 4

Ingredients:
- 1½ lb tofu halved lengthwise
- Salt and ground black pepper to taste
- 2 eggs
- 2 tbsp Italian seasoning
- 1 pinch red chili flakes
- ½ cup sliced Pecorino Romano cheese
- ¼ cup fresh parsley, chopped
- 4 tbsp butter
- 2 garlic cloves, minced
- 2 cups crushed tomatoes
- 1 tbsp dried basil
- Salt and ground black pepper to taste
- ½ lb sliced mozzarella cheese

Directions:
- Preheat the oven to 400 F and grease a baking dish with cooking spray. Set aside.
- Season the tofu with salt and black pepper; set aside.

- In a medium bowl, whisk the eggs with the Italian seasoning, and red chili flakes. On a plate, combine the Pecorino Romano cheese with parsley.
- Melt the butter in a medium skillet over medium heat.
- Quickly dip the tofu in the egg mixture and then dredge generously in the cheese mixture.
- Place in the butter and fry on both sides until the cheese melts and is golden brown, 8 to 10 minutes. Place on a plate and set aside.
- Sauté the garlic in the same pan and mix in the tomatoes. Top with the basil, salt, and black pepper, and cook for 5 to 10 minutes. Pour the sauce into the baking dish.
- Lay the tofu pieces in the sauce and top with the mozzarella cheese. Bake in the oven for 10 to 15 minutes or until the cheese melts completely.
- Remove the dish and serve with a leafy green salad.

Nutrition:
Calories:140 | Total Fat:13.2g | Saturated Fat:7.1g | Total Carbs:2g | Dietary Fiber:0g | Sugar:0g | Protein:3g | Sodium:78 mg

Seitan Meatza with Kale

Preparation Time: 10minutes | Cooking Time: 22minutes | Servings: 4

Ingredients:

- 1 lb ground seitan
- Salt and black pepper to taste
- 2 cups powdered Parmesan cheese
- ¼ tsp onion powder
- ¼ tsp garlic powder
- ½ cup unsweetened tomato sauce
- 1 tsp white vinegar
- ½ tsp liquid smoke
- ¼ cup baby kale, chopped roughly
- 1 cup mozzarella cheese

Directions:

- Preheat the oven to 400 F and line a medium pizza pan with parchment paper and grease with cooking spray. Set aside.

- In a medium bowl, combine the seitan, salt, black pepper, and parmesan cheese. Spread the mixture on the pizza pan to fit the shape of the pan. Bake in the oven for 15 minutes or until the meat cooks.

- Meanwhile in a medium bowl, mix the onion powder, garlic powder, tomato sauce, vinegar, and liquid smoke. Remove the meat crust from the oven and spread the tomato mixture on top. Add the kale and sprinkle with the mozzarella cheese.

- Bake in the oven for 7 minutes or until the cheese melts.

- Take out from the oven, slice, and serve warm.

Nutrition:

Calories:601 | Total Fat:51.8g | Saturated Fat:16.4g | Total Carbs:18g | Dietary Fiber:5g | Sugar:3g | Protein:23g | Sodium:398mg

Broccoli Tempeh

Preparation Time: 10minutes | Cooking Time: 15minutes | Servings: 4

Ingredients:

- 6 slices tempeh, chopped
- 2 tbsp butter
- 4 tofu, cut into 1-inch cubes
- Salt and ground black pepper to taste
- 4 garlic cloves, minced
- 1 cup baby kale, chopped
- 1 ½ cups full- fat heavy cream
- 1 medium head broccoli, cut into florets
- ¼ cup shredded parmesan cheese

Directions:

- Put the tempeh in a medium skillet over medium heat and fry until crispy and brown, 5 minutes. Spoon onto a plate and set aside.

- Melt the butter in the same skillet, season the tofu with salt and black pepper, and cook on both sides until golden- brown. Spoon onto the tempeh's plate and set aside.

- Add the garlic to the skillet, sauté for 1 minute.

- Mix in the full- fat heavy cream, tofu, and tempeh, and kale, allow simmering for 5 minutes or until the sauce thickens.

- Meanwhile, pour the broccoli into a large safe-microwave bowl, sprinkle with some water, season with salt, and black pepper, and microwave for 2 minutes or until the broccoli softens.

- Spoon the broccoli into the sauce, top with the parmesan cheese, stir and cook until the cheese melts. Turn the heat off.

- Spoon the mixture into a serving platter and serve warm.

Nutrition:

Calories:193 | Total Fat:20.1g | Saturated Fat:12.5g | Total Carbs:3g | Dietary Fiber:0g | Sugar:2g | Protein:1g | Sodium:100mg

Avocado Seitan

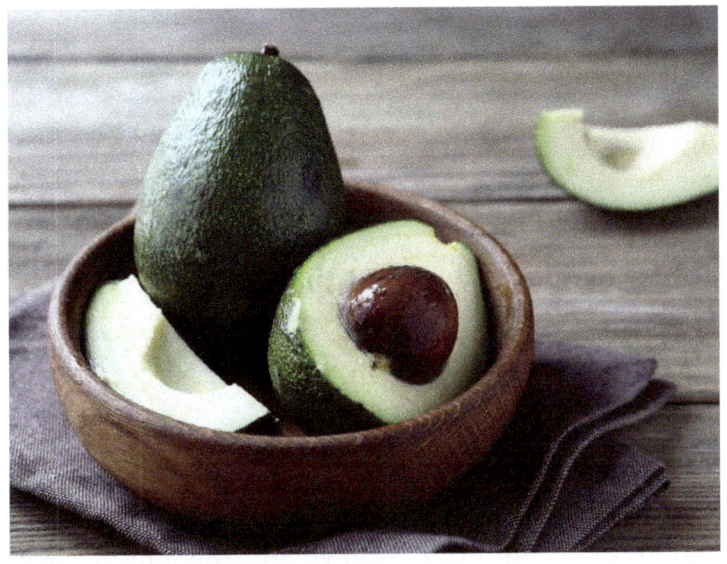

Preparation Time: 10 minutes | Cooking Time: 2 hours 15 minutes | Servings: 4

Ingredients:

- 1 white onion, finely chopped
- ¼ cup vegetable stock
- 3 tbsp coconut oil
- 3 tbsp tamari sauce
- 3 tbsp chili pepper
- 1 tbsp red wine vinegar

- Salt and ground black pepper to taste
- 2 lb Seitan
- 1 large avocado, halved and pitted
- ½ lemon, juiced

Directions:

- In a large pot, combine the onion, vegetable stock, coconut oil, tamari sauce, chili pepper, red wine vinegar, salt, black pepper. Add the seitan, close the lid, and cook over low heat for 2 hours.
- Scoop the avocado pulp into a bowl, add the lemon juice, and using a fork, mash the avocado into a puree. Set aside.
- When ready, turn the heat off and mix in the avocado. Adjust the taste with salt and black pepper.
- Spoon onto a serving platter and serve warm.

Nutrition:

Calories:412 | Total Fat:43g | Saturated Fat:37g | Total Carbs:9g | Dietary Fiber:3g | Sugar:0g | Protein:5g | Sodium:12mg

Jamaican Jerk Tempeh

Preparation Time: 15 minutes | Cooking Time: 45 minutes | Servings: 4

Ingredients:

- ½ cup plain unsweetened yogurt
- 2 tbsp melted butter
- 2 tbsp Jamaican jerk seasoning
- Salt and black pepper to taste
- 2 lb tempeh
- 3 tbsp tofu
- ¼ cup almond meal

Directions:

- Preheat the oven to 350 F and grease a baking sheet with cooking spray.
- In a large bowl, combine the plain yogurt, butter, Jamaican jerk seasoning, salt, and black

pepper. Add the tempeh and toss to coat evenly. Allow marinating for 15 minutes.

- In a food processor, blend the tofu with the almond meal until finely combined. Pour the mixture onto a wide plate.

- Remove the tempeh from the marinade, shake off any excess liquid, and coat generously in the tofu mixture. Place on the baking sheet and grease lightly with cooking spray.

- Bake in the oven for 40 to 45 minutes or until golden brown and crispy, turning once.

- Remove the tempeh and serve warm with red cabbage slaw and parsnip fries.

Nutrition:

Calories:684 | Total Fat:68g | Saturated Fat:12.1g | Total Carbs:13g | Dietary Fiber:4g | Sugar:1g | Protein:13g | Sodium:653mg

Curried Tofu Meatballs

Preparation Time: 5 minutes | Cooking Time: 25 minutes | Servings: 4

Ingredients:

- 3 lb ground tofu
- 1 medium yellow onion, finely chopped
- 2 green bell peppers, deseeded and chopped
- 3 garlic cloves, minced
- 2 tbsp melted butter
- 1 tsp dried parsley
- 2 tbsp hot sauce
- Salt and ground black pepper to taste
- 1 tbsp red curry powder
- 3 tbsp olive oil

Directions:

• Preheat the oven to 400 F and grease a baking sheet with cooking spray.

• In a bowl, combine the tofu, onion, bell peppers, garlic, butter, parsley, hot sauce, salt, black pepper, and curry powder. With your hands, form a 1-inch tofu ball from the mixture and place it on the greased baking sheet.

• Drizzle the olive oil over the meat and bake in the oven until the tofu balls are brown on the outside and cook within, 20 to 25 minutes.

• Remove the dish from the oven and plate the tofu ball.

• Garnish with some scallions and serve warm on a bed of spinach salad with herbed vegan paneer cheese dressing.

Nutrition:

Calories:506 | Total Fat:45.6g | Saturated Fat:18.9g | Total Carbs:11g | Dietary Fiber:1g | Sugar:1g | Protein:19g | Sodium:794mg

Spicy Mushroom Collard Wraps

Preparation Time: 10 minutes | Cooking Time: 16 minutes | Servings: 4

Ingredients:

- 2 tbsp avocado oil
- 1 large yellow onion, chopped
- 2 garlic cloves, minced
- Salt and ground black pepper to taste
- 1 small jalapeño pepper, deseeded and finely chopped
- 1 ½ lb mushrooms, cut into 1-inch cubes
- 1 cup cauliflower rice
- 2 tsp hot sauce
- 8 collard leaves
- ¼ cup plain unsweetened yogurt for topping

Directions:

- Heat 2 tablespoons of avocado oil in a large deep skillet; add and sauté the onion until softened, 3 minutes.

- Pour in the garlic, salt, black pepper, and jalapeño pepper; cook until fragrant, 1 minute.

- Mix in the mushrooms and cook both sides, 10 minutes.

- Add the cauliflower rice and hot sauce. Sauté until the cauliflower slightly softens, 2 to 3 minutes. Adjust the taste with salt and black pepper.

- Lay the collards on a clean flat surface and spoon the curried mixture onto the middle part of the leaves, about 3 tablespoons per leaf. Spoon the plain yogurt on top, wrap the leaves, and serve immediately.

Nutrition:

Calories:380 | Total Fat:34.8g | Saturated Fat:19.9g | Total Carbs:10g | Dietary Fiber:5g | Sugar:5g | Protein:10g | Sodium:395mg

Pesto Tofu Zoodles

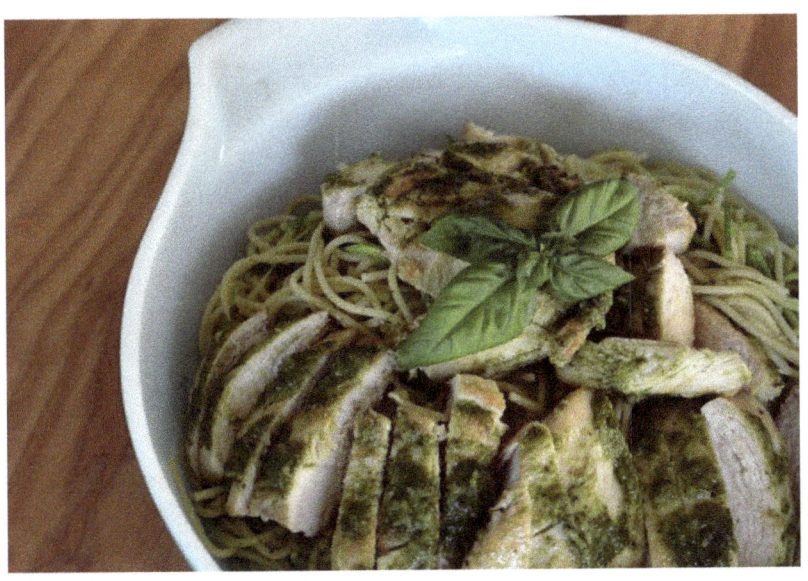

Preparation Time: 5minutes | Cooking Time: 12minutes | Servings: 4

Ingredients:

- 2 tbsp olive oil
- 1 medium white onion, chopped
- 1 garlic clove, minced
- 2 (14 oz blocks firm tofu, pressed and cubed
- 1 medium red bell pepper, deseeded and sliced

- 6 medium zucchinis, spiralized
- Salt and black pepper to taste
- ¼ cup basil pesto, olive oil-based
- 2/3 cup grated parmesan cheese
- ½ cup shredded mozzarella cheese
- Toasted pine nuts to garnish

Directions:

- Heat the olive oil in a medium pot over medium heat; sauté the onion and garlic until softened and fragrant, 3 minutes.

- Add the tofu and cook until golden on all sides then pour in the bell pepper and cook until softened, 4 minutes.

- Mix in the zucchinis, pour the pesto on top, and season with salt and black pepper. Cook for 3 to 4 minutes or until the zucchinis soften a little bit. Turn the heat off and carefully stir in the parmesan cheese.

- Dish into four plates, share the mozzarella cheese on top, garnish with the pine nuts, and serve warm.

Nutrition:

Calories:79 | Total Fat:6.2g | Saturated Fat:3.7g | Total Carbs:5g | Dietary Fiber:2g | Sugar:3g | Protein:2g | Sodium:54mg

Cheesy Mushroom Pie

Preparation Time: 12minutes | Cooking Time: 43minutes | Servings: 4

Ingredients:

For the pie crust:

- ¼ cup almond flour + extra for dusting

- 3 tbsp coconut flour

- ½ tsp salt

- ¼ cup butter, cold and crumbled

- 3 tbsp erythritol

- 1 ½ tsp vanilla extract

- 4 whole eggs

For the filling:

- 2 tbsp butter

- 1 medium yellow onion

- 2 garlic cloves, minced

- 2 cups mixed mushrooms, chopped

- 1 green bell pepper, deseeded and diced

- 1 cup green beans, cut into 3 pieces each

- Salt and black pepper to taste

- ¼ cup coconut cream

- 1/3 cup vegan sour cream

- ½ cup almond milk

- 2 eggs, lightly beaten

- ¼ tsp nutmeg powder

- 1 tbsp chopped parsley

- 1 cup grated parmesan cheese

Directions:

For the pastry crust:

- Preheat the oven to 350 F and grease a pie pan with cooking spray

- In a large bowl, mix the almond flour, coconut flour, and salt.

- Add the butter and mix with an electric hand mixer until crumbly. Add the erythritol and vanilla extract until mixed in. Then, pour in the eggs one after another while mixing until formed into a ball.

- Flatten the dough on a clean flat surface, cover in plastic wrap, and refrigerate for 1 hour.

- After, lightly dust a clean flat surface with almond flour, unwrap the dough, and roll out the dough into a large rectangle, ½ - inch thickness and fit into a pie pan.

- Pour some baking beans onto the pastry and bake in the oven until golden. Remove after, pour the beans, and allow cooling.

For the filling:

- Meanwhile, melt the butter in a skillet and sauté the onion and garlic until softened and fragrant, 3 minutes. Add the mushrooms, bell pepper, green beans, salt, and black pepper; cook for 5 minutes.

- In a medium bowl, beat the coconut cream, vegan sour cream, milk, and eggs. Season with black pepper, salt, and nutmeg. Stir in the parsley and cheese.

- Spread the mushroom mixture in the baked pastry and spread the cheese filling on top. Place the pie in the oven and bake for 30 to 35 minutes or until a toothpick inserted into the pie comes out clean and golden on top.

- Remove, let cool for 10 minutes, slice, and serve with roasted tomato salad.

Nutrition:

Calories:120 | Total Fat:9.2g | Saturated Fat:2.3g | Total Carbs:7g | Dietary Fiber:3g | Sugar:3g | Protein:5g | Sodium:17mg

Tofu Scallopini with Lemon

Preparation Time: 5minutes | Cooking Time: 21minutes | Servings: 4

Ingredients:

- 1½ lb thin cut tofu chops, boneless
- Salt and ground black pepper to taste
- 1 tbsp avocado oil
- 3 tbsp butter
- 2 tbsp capers
- 1 cup vegetable broth
- ½ lemon, juiced + 1 lemon, sliced
- 2 tbsp freshly chopped parsley

Directions:

- Heat the avocado oil in a large skillet over medium heat. Season the tofu chops with salt and black pepper; cook in the oil on both sides until brown and cooked through 12 to 15 minutes. Transfer to a plate, cover with another plate and keep warm.

- Add the butter to the pan to melt and cook the capers until hot and sizzling stirring frequently to avoid burning for 3 minutes.

- Pour in the vegetable broth and lemon juice, use a spatula to scrape any bits stuck to the bottom of the pan, and allow boiling until the sauce reduces by half.

- Add the tofu back to the sauce, arrange the lemon slices on top, and sprinkle with half of the parsley. Allow simmering for 3 minutes.

- Plate the food, garnish with the remaining parsley, and serve warm with creamy mashed cauliflower.

Nutrition:

Calories:214 | Total Fat:15.6g | Saturated Fat:2.5g | Total Carbs:12g | Dietary Fiber:2g | Sugar:6g | Protein:9g | Sodium:280mg

Tofu Chops with Green Beans and Avocado Sauté

Preparation Time: 10minutes | Cooking Time: 22 minutes | Servings: 4

Ingredients:

For the tofu chops:

- 2 tbsp avocado oil
- 4 slices firm tofu
- Salt and ground black pepper to taste

For the green beans and avocado sauté:

- 2 tbsp avocado oil
- 1 ½ cups green beans
- 2 large avocados, halved, pitted, and chopped
- Salt and ground black pepper to taste
- 6 green onions, chopped
- 1 tbsp freshly chopped parsley

Directions:

For the tofu chops:

- Heat the avocado oil in a medium skillet, season the tofu with salt and black pepper, and fry

in the oil on both sides until brown, and cooked through for 12 to 15 minutes. Transfer to a plate and set aside in a warmer for serving.

For the green beans and avocado sauté:

- Heat the avocado oil in a medium skillet, add and sauté the green beans until sweating and slightly softened for 10 minutes. Mix in the avocados (don't worry if they mash up a bit), season with salt and black pepper, and half of the green onions. Warm the avocados for 2 minutes. Turn the heat off.

- Dish the sauté into serving plates, garnish with the remaining green onions and parsley, and serve with the tofu chops.

Nutrition:

Calories:503 | Total Fat:41.9g | Saturated Fat:14.5g | Total Carbs:18g | Dietary Fiber:2g | Sugar:4g | Protein:19g | Sodium:314mg

Mushroom in Tortillas

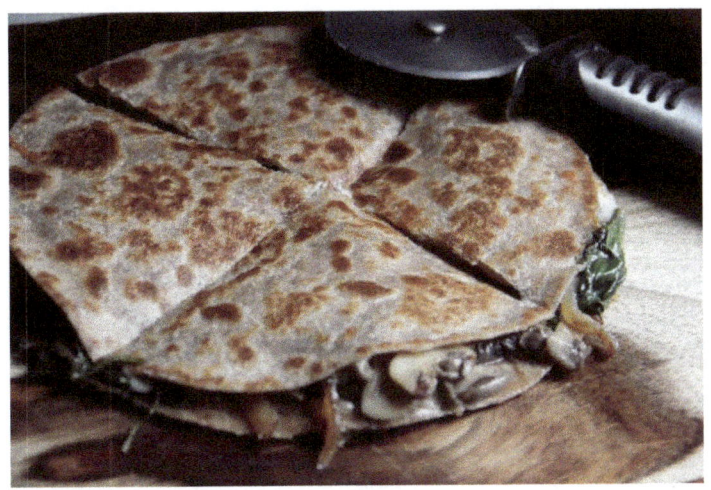

Preparation Time: 15minutes | Cooking Time: 6hours, 64minutes | Servings: 4

Ingredients:

For the mushrooms:

- 2 tbsp olive oil

- ½ cup sliced yellow onion

- 2 lb mushroom

- 4 tbsp ras el hanout seasoning

- Salt to taste

- 3 ½ cups vegetable broth

For the keto tortillas:

- 5 tbsp psyllium husk powder
- 1¼ cups almond flour
- 1 tsp salt
- 2 eggs, cracked into a bowl
- 1 cup of water
- 2 tbsp butter, for frying

Directions:

For the mushroom:

- In a large pot, heat the olive oil and sauté the onion for 3 minutes or until softened. Season the mushrooms with ras el hanout, salt, and place in the onion. Sear on each side for 3 minutes and pour the vegetable broth on top. Cover the lid, reduce the heat to low, and cook for 4 to 5 hours or until the mushroom softens.

- After, open the lid and shred the mushroom with two forks. Cook further over low heat for 1 hour to allow the spices to penetrate the meat strands. Turn the heat off and using a slotted spoon, transfer the meat onto a plate. Set aside in a warmer for serving.

For the keto tortillas:

- In a medium bowl, combine the psyllium husk powder, almond flour, and salt. Mix in the eggs until a thick dough forms and then the water. Separate the dough into 8 or 10 pieces. • Lay a parchment paper on a flat surface, grease with a little cooking spray, and put a dough piece on top. Cover with another parchment paper and, using a rolling pin, flatten the dough into a circle. Repeat the same process for the remaining dough balls.

- Melt a quarter of the butter in a large skillet over medium heat and fry the flattened dough one after another on both sides until light brown and cooked through, 40 minutes in total.

- Transfer the keto tortillas to serving plates, spoon the shredded meat onto the keto tortillas and top with some leafy greens. Serve immediately.

Nutrition:

Calories:345 | Total Fat:26.1g | Saturated Fat:15.4g | Total Carbs:11g | Dietary Fiber:5g | Sugar:5g | Protein:20g | Sodium:402mg

Hazelnuts and Cheese Stuffed Zucchinis

Preparation Time: 15minutes | Cooking Time: 20minutes | Servings: 4

Ingredients:

- 2 tbsp olive oil
- 1 cup cauliflower rice
- ¼ cup vegetable broth
- 1 ¼ cup diced tomatoes
- 1 medium red onion, chopped
- ¼ cup pine nuts
- ¼ cup hazelnuts
- 4 tbsp chopped cilantro
- 1 tbsp balsamic vinegar
- 1 tbsp smoked paprika
- 4 medium zucchinis, halved
- 1 cup grated parmesan cheese

Directions:

- Preheat the oven to 350 F.

- Pour the cauliflower rice and vegetable broth into a medium pot and cook over medium heat for 5 minutes or until softened. Turn the heat off, fluff the cauliflower rice, and allow cooling.

- Scoop the flesh out of the zucchini halves using a spoon and chop the pulp. Brush the inner parts of the vegetable with olive oil.

- In a bowl, mix the cauliflower rice, tomatoes, red onion, pine nuts, hazelnuts, cilantro, balsamic vinegar, paprika, zucchini pulp, salt, and black pepper.

- Spoon the mixture into the zucchini halves, drizzle with more olive oil, and sprinkle the cheese on top.

- Place the stuffed vegetables on a baking sheet and bake in the oven for 15 to 20 minutes or until the cheese has melted and golden.

- Remove, allow cooling, and serve.

Nutrition:

Calories:197 | Total Fat:15.6g | Saturated Fat:9.3g | Total Carbs:5g | Dietary Fiber:0g | Sugar:1g | Protein:9g | Sodium:1179mg

Tempeh Stuffed Mushrooms

Preparation Time: 5minutes | Cooking Time: 20minutes | Servings: 4

Ingredients:

- 2 tbsp butter
- ½ lb ground tempeh
- Salt and ground black pepper to taste
- 1 tsp paprika
- 3 tbsp fresh chives, finely chopped
- 7 oz cashew cream
- 12 medium portabella mushrooms, stalks removed
- ¼ cup shredded Soy cheese

Directions:

- Preheat the oven to 400 F and grease a baking sheet with cooking spray. Set aside.

- Melt the butter in a medium skillet over medium heat; add the tempeh, season with salt, black pepper, and paprika. Cook until brown, 10 minutes while frequently stirring to break any lumps that form. Turn the heat off and mix in two-thirds of the chives and all the cashew cream until evenly combined.

- Place the mushrooms on the baking sheet and spoon the mixture into the mushrooms. Top with the Soy cheese and bake in the oven until the mushrooms turn golden and the cheese melted, 10 minutes.

- Remove the stuffed mushrooms onto serving plates, garnish with the remaining chives, and serve immediately.

Nutrition:

Calories:159 | Total Fat:14.6g | Saturated Fat:7.9g | Total Carbs:3g | Dietary Fiber:0g | Sugar:0g | Protein:5g | Sodium:94mg

Mushroom and Vegan Bacon Lettuce Wraps

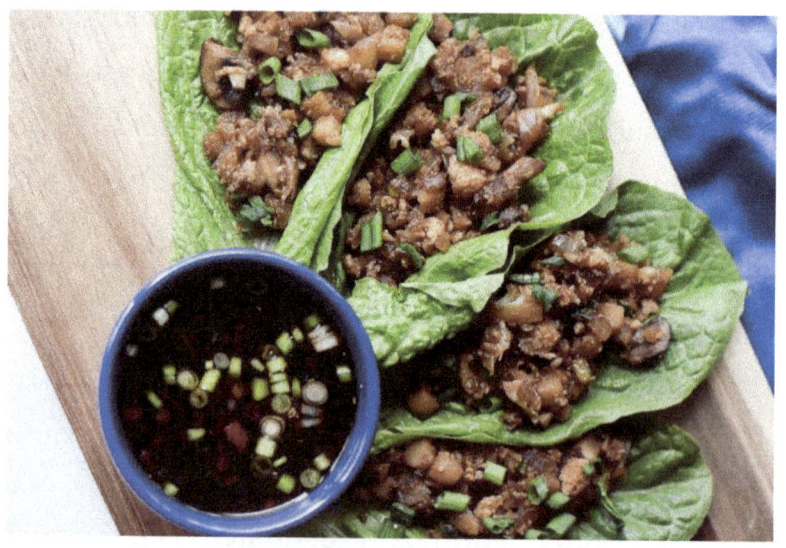

Preparation Time: 10minutes | Cooking Time: 15minutes | Servings: 4

Ingredients:

- 8 vegan bacon slices, chopped

- 2 tbsp olive oil

- ½ cup sliced cremini mushrooms

- Salt and ground black pepper to taste

- 1½ lb crumbled tempeh

- 1 iceberg lettuce, leaves separated and washed
- 1 cup shredded cheddar cheese

Directions:

- In a large skillet, add the bacon and cook over medium heat until brown and crispy. Transfer onto a paper-towel-lined plate and set aside.

- Add 1 tablespoon of olive oil to the skillet to heat and sauté the mushrooms. Season with salt and black pepper; allow cooking for 5 minutes or until softened.

- Add the remaining oil to the skillet to heat and cook the tempeh (season with salt and black pepper until brown, 10 minutes, while breaking the lumps that form. Turn the heat off.

- Divide the tempeh into the lettuce leaves, sprinkle with the cheddar cheese, top with the vegan bacon and mushrooms. Wrap the leaves and serve immediately with mayonnaise.

Nutrition:

Calories:447 | Total Fat:43.6g | Saturated Fat:26.4g | Total Carbs:13g | Dietary Fiber:1g | Sugar:0g | Protein:10g | Sodium:1403mg

Mushroom in Thai Curry Sauce

Preparation Time: 15minutes | Cooking Time: 25minutes, 30seconds | Servings: 4

Ingredients:

- 6 tbsp butter

- 1 medium canon cabbage, shredded

- Salt and ground black pepper to taste

- 1 lb mushrooms

- 1 celery, chopped

- 1 tbsp red curry powder

- 1 ¼ cups coconut cream

Directions:

- Melt 2 tablespoons of butter in a medium skillet, add and sauté the cabbage until soft and slightly golden, and season with salt and black pepper, 5 minutes. Spoon the cabbage onto a plate and set aside.

- Melt 2 tablespoons of butter in the skillet, season the mushroom with salt and black pepper, and fry in the fat until brown on the outside and cooked within, 10 minutes. Remove onto a plate and set aside.

- Add the remaining butter to the skillet and once melted, sauté the celery until softened. Mix in the curry powder, heat for 30 seconds, and stir in the coconut cream. Allow simmering for 5 to 10 minutes. Season with salt and black pepper.

- Put the meat in the sauce and spoon some sauce over the mushroom. Turn the heat off.

- Serve the mushroom and curry sauce with the buttered cabbage.

Nutrition:

Calories:310 | Total Fat:24.5g | Saturated Fat:11.8g | Total Carbs:10g | Dietary Fiber:2g | Sugar:5g | Protein:16g | Sodium:136mg

Baked Camembert Cheese with Seitan and Pecans

Preparation Time: 8minutes | Cooking Time: 22minutes | Servings: 4

Ingredients:

- 9 oz whole Camembert cheese
- 3 tbsp olive oil
- ½ lb seitan chops, cut into small cubes
- Salt and ground black pepper to taste
- 2 oz pecans
- 1 garlic clove, minced
- 1 tbsp freshly chopped parsley

Directions:

- Preheat the oven to 400 F.
- While the cheese is in its box, using a knife, score around the top and side of about a ¼ -inch into the cheese and take off the top layer of the skin.

- Place the cheese on a baking tray and melt in the oven for 8 to 10 minutes.

- Remove the cheese from the oven after.

- For the topping:

- Meanwhile, heat the olive oil in a medium skillet over medium heat, season the seitan with salt and black pepper, and fry in the oil until brown on all sides with a little crust, 10 to 12 minutes. Transfer to a medium mixing bowl and add the pecans, garlic, and parsley.

- Spoon the mixture onto the cheese and bake in the oven for 10 minutes or until the cheese softens and nuts toasts.

- Serve warm with low carb bread or steamed asparagus.

Nutrition:

Calories:266 | Total Fat:24.9g | Saturated Fat:4.7g | Total Carbs:6g | Dietary Fiber:1g | Sugar:2g | Protein:7g | Sodium:232mg

Cheesy Tempeh Burrito Bowl

Preparation Time: 10minutes | Cooking Time: 15minutes | Servings: 4

Ingredients:

- 1 tbsp butter

- 1 lb ground tempeh

- ½ cup vegetable broth

- 4 tbsp taco seasoning

- Salt and ground black pepper to taste

- ½ cup sharp cheddar cheese, shredded

- ½ cup sour cream

- ¼ cup sliced black olives

- 1 avocado, cubed

- ¼ cup tomatoes, diced

- 1 green onion, sliced

- 1 tbsp fresh cilantro, chopped

Directions:

- Melt the butter in a large skillet over medium heat. Add and cook the tempeh until brown while breaking any lumps that form, 10 minutes.

- Mix in the vegetable broth, taco seasoning, salt, and black pepper; cook until most of the liquid has evaporated, 5 minutes.

- Mix in half of the cheddar cheese and allow melting. Turn the heat off.

- Spoon the dish into a large serving bowl and top with olives, avocado, tomatoes, green onion, and cilantro.

- Serve warm with low carb tortillas.

Nutrition:

Calories:530 |, Total Fat:57.5g | Saturated Fat:8.9g | Total Carbs:3g | Dietary Fiber:1g | Sugar:1g | Protein:3g | Sodium:8mg

Tofu Casserole with Cottage Cheese

Preparation Time: 5 minutes | Cooking Time: 5 minutes | Servings: 4

Ingredients:

- 2 tbsp avocado oil
- 1½ lb crumbled tofu
- Salt and black pepper to taste
- ¼ cup sliced Kalamata olives
- ½ cup cottage cheese, crumbled
- 2 garlic cloves, minced
- ½ cup unsweetened marinara sauce
- 1 ¼ cups heavy cream

Directions:

- Preheat the oven to 400 F and lightly grease a casserole dish with cooking spray. Set aside.

- Heat the avocado oil in a deep, medium skillet over medium heat, add the tofu, season with salt and black pepper, and cook until brown, 10 minutes. Stir frequently.

- Transfer and spread the tofu in the bottom of the casserole dish. Scatter the olives, cottage cheese, and garlic on top.

- In a medium bowl, mix the marinara sauce and heavy cream, and pour the mixture all over the other Ingredients.

- Bake in the oven until the top is bubbly and lightly brown, 20 to 30 minutes.

- Remove after and dish into serving plates.

- Serve warm with a leafy green salad.

Nutrition:

Calories:511 | Total Fat:46.4g | Saturated Fat:7.5g | Total Carbs:13g | Dietary Fiber:4g | Sugar:5g | Protein:16g | Sodium:153mg

Egg Roll and Tofu Bowl

Preparation Time: 15minutes | Cooking Time: 15minutes | Servings: 4

Ingredients:

- 2 tbsp sesame oil
- 2 large eggs
- 2 tbsp minced garlic
- ½ tsp ginger puree
- 1 medium white onion, diced
- 1 lb ground tofu
- Salt and ground black pepper to taste
- 1 habanero pepper, chopped
- 1 small green cabbage, shredded
- 5 scallions, chopped
- 3 tbsp coconut aminos
- 1 tbsp white vinegar
- 2 tbsp sesame seeds

Directions:

- Heat 1 tablespoon of sesame oil in a medium skillet over medium heat and scramble the eggs until set, 1 minute. Transfer to a plate and set aside.

- Heat the remaining sesame oil in the same skillet and sauté the garlic, ginger, and onion in the same skillet until softened and fragrant, 4 minutes.

- Add the ground tofu, season with salt, black pepper, and habanero pepper. Cook until the tofu turns brown, 10 minutes.

- Mix in the cabbage, scallions, coconut aminos, and vinegar and cook until the cabbage is tender. Stir in the eggs and adjust the taste with salt and black pepper.

- Dish the food, garnish with the sesame seeds and serve with low carb tortillas.

Nutrition:

Calories:319 | Total Fat:23.1g | Saturated Fat:13.4g | Total Carbs:7g | Dietary Fiber:2g | Sugar:4g | Protein:21g | Sodium:1060mg

Pizza Alla Puttanesca

Preparation Time: 15 minutes | Cooking Time: 30-120 minutes | Servings: 6

Ingredients:

Dough:

- 1½ cups unbleached all-purpose flour
- ½ cup warm water, or as needed
- 1 tablespoon olive oil
- 1½ teaspoons instant yeast
- ½ teaspoon salt
- ½ teaspoon Italian seasoning

Sauce:

- ½ cup crushed tomatoes
- ½ cup shredded vegan mozzarella cheese
- ¼ cup pitted green olives, sliced
- ¼ cup pitted kalamata olives, sliced
- 1 tablespoon chopped fresh flat-leaf parsley

- 1 tablespoon capers, rinsed and drained
- ¼ teaspoon garlic powder
- ¼ teaspoon sugar
- ¼ teaspoon dried basil
- ¼ teaspoon dried oregano
- ¼ teaspoon hot red pepper flakes
- Salt and freshly ground black pepper

Directions:

- Get a bowl to mix your dough. Whisk together the flour, yeast, salt, and seasoning.

- Add the oil slowly whilst stirring, then add water little by little until the dough ball is formed.

- Knead the dough on a floured surface for 2 minutes.

- Shape it and put it in a warm bowl to rise for an hour.

- Whilst the dough rises, mix the sauce. Combine tomatoes, olives, capers, parsley, basil, oregano, garlic powder, sugar, red pepper, salt, and pepper.

- Oil a tray that will fit in your Pressure pot and stretch the dough to fit it.

- Spread the sauce over the dough.

- Insert the tray into your Pressure pot and cook for 10 minutes on steam.

- Release the pressure quickly and sprinkle the mozzarella on top at the end.

Nutrition:

Calories:680 | Total Fat:71.8g | Saturated Fat:20.9g | Total Carbs:10g | Dietary Fiber:7g | Sugar:2g | Protein:3g | Sodium:525mg

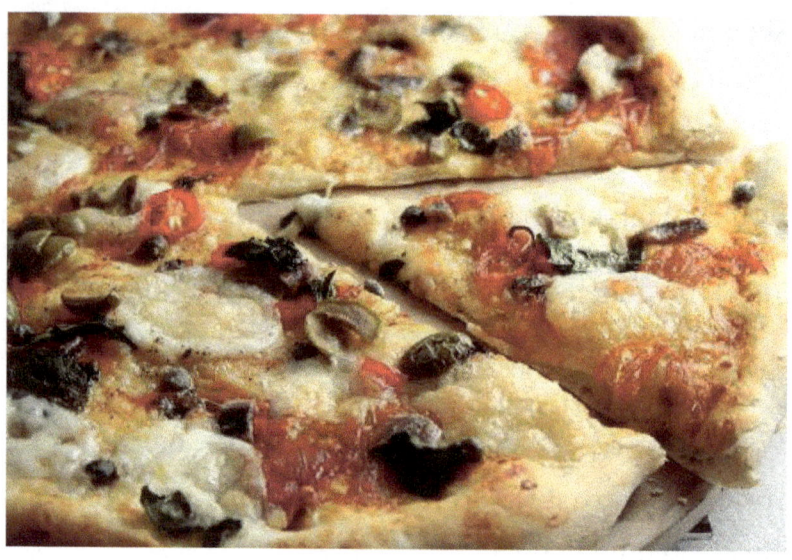

Seitan Fajitas

Preparation Time: 40 minutes | Cooking Time: 30-120 minutes | Servings: 6

Ingredients:

- 1lb seitan, cut into strips
- 2 tablespoons tomato paste
- 1½ cups tomato salsa
- 1 tablespoon chili powder
- 1 tablespoon soy sauce
- 2 large bell peppers (any color), seeded and cut into ¼-inch-thick strips
- 1 large yellow onion, thinly sliced
- 1 garlic clove, minced
- Salt and freshly ground black pepper
- 2 tablespoons freshly squeezed lime juice
- 1 ripe Hass avocado, peeled, pitted, and diced, for garnish
- 1 large ripe tomato, diced, for garnish

Directions:

- Mix the tomato paste, salsa, chili powder, and soy sauce until combined well.

- Put the bell peppers, onion, and garlic in your Pressure pot.

- Put your seitan strips on top. Try and avoid touching them.

- Pour the tomato mix over everything.

- Seal and cook on Poultry for 30 minutes.

- Depressurize naturally, stir in the lime to taste.

- Serve and top with avocado and tomato.

Nutrition:

Calories: 140 Cal | Fat: 0.9 g | Carbs: 27.1 g | Protein: 6.3 g | Fiber: 6.2 g

Zesty Stuffed Bell Peppers

Preparation Time: 30 minutes | Cooking Time: 30-120 minutes | Servings: 4

Ingredients:

• 4 large bell peppers (any color or a combination

• 1 (14-ounce can tomato sauce

• 2 cups cooked brown or white rice

• 1½ cups cooked pinto beans or black beans or 1 (15-ounce) can beans, rinsed and drained

• 1 cup fresh or thawed frozen corn kernels

• 1 cup diced fresh tomatoes or 1 (14-ounce can diced tomatoes, drained

• 2 teaspoons olive oil (optional

• 4 garlic cloves, minced

• 4 scallions, chopped

• 1 tablespoon chili powder

• 2 teaspoons minced chipotle chiles in adobo

• 1½ teaspoon ground cumin

• 1¼ teaspoon dried oregano

- ½ teaspoon sugar

- Salt and freshly ground black pepper

Directions:

- Warm the oil in your Pressure pot, leaving the lid open.

- When the oil is hot, add the garlic and scallions and soften for 3 minutes.

- Add the chili powder and a teaspoon of both the cumin and the oregano.

- Put the garlic mixture in a bowl to one side. Add the rice, beans, corn, tomatoes, and chiles with a little salt and pepper. Mix well.

- Top and hollow your bell peppers.

- Fill the peppers evenly with the mix and set them in the steamer basket of your Pressure pot. • Mix the tomato sauce, remaining cumin, remaining oregano, sugar, and salt in the base of your Pressure pot.

- Lower the steamer basket, seal, and cook on Steam for 24 minutes.

- Depressurize fast and serve immediately.

Nutrition:

Calories: 140 Cal | Fat: 0.9 g | Carbs: 27.1 g | Protein: 6.3 g | Fiber: 6.2 g

Moroccan Stuffed Peppers

Preparation Time: 30 minutes | Cooking Time: 30-120 minutes | Servings: 4

Ingredients:

- 4 large bell peppers (assorted colors look great
- 2 cups boiling water or vegetable broth
- 2 cups couscous
- 1 cup cooked chickpeas or 1 (15-ounce can chickpeas
- 1 medium-size yellow onion, minced
- 2 carrots, peeled and minced
- 1 large zucchini, minced
- 3 garlic cloves, minced
- 3 tablespoons tomato paste
- 2 teaspoons olive oil
- 2 teaspoons harissa or hot chili paste
- 2 teaspoons ground coriander
- 1 teaspoon paprika
- 1 teaspoon ground cinnamon
- ½ tablespoon ground cumin
- 1 teaspoon salt
- ¼ teaspoon freshly ground black pepper

- 1 tablespoon minced fresh flat-leaf parsley leaves, for garnish

Directions:

- Top and hollow the peppers. Remove the stems, then chop the tops and keep the diced pepper.

- Warm the oil in your Pressure pot.

- When hot, add the onion and soften for 4 minutes.

- Add the carrots, pepper tops, zucchini, garlic, and cook for 2 more minutes.

- Add the harissa, tomato paste, coriander, cinnamon, cumin, paprika, salt, and pepper.

- Add the couscous and water, stir well.

- Add the chickpeas and stir again.

- Pack the stuffing into the peppers and put them in the steamer basket of your Pressure pot.

- Put a cup of water in your Pressure pot. Lower the steamer basket.

- Seal and cook on Steam for 24 minutes.

- Depressurize naturally and serve immediately, topped with parsley.

Nutrition:

Calories:680 | Total Fat:71.8g | Saturated Fat:20.9g | Total Carbs:10g | Dietary Fiber:7g | Sugar:2g | Protein:3g | Sodium:525mg

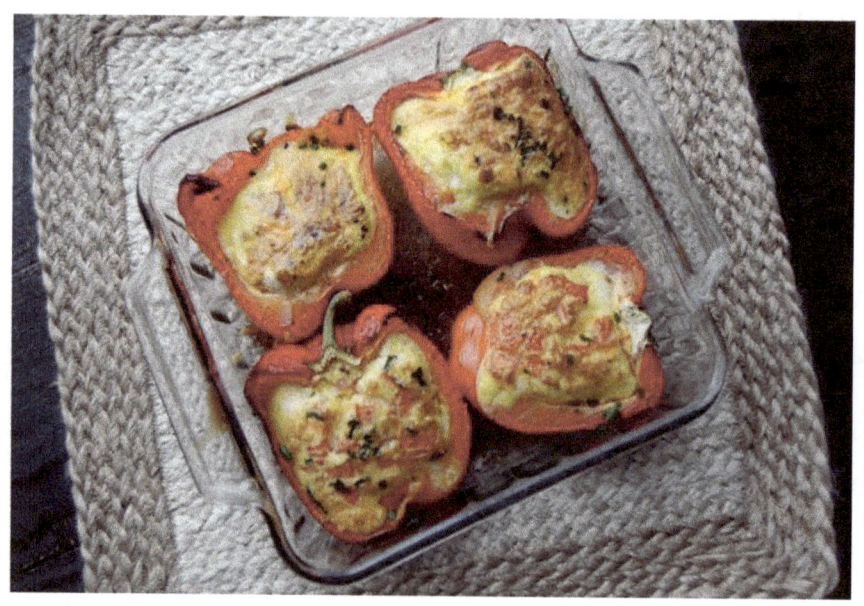

Tempeh Chops with Caramelized Onions and Brie Cheese

Preparation Time: 10minutes | Cooking Time: 35minutes | Servings: 4

Ingredients:

- 3 tbsp olive oil
- 2 large red onions, sliced
- 2 tbsp balsamic vinegar
- 1 tsp sugar-free maple syrup
- Salt and ground black pepper to taste
- 4 mushroom chops
- 4 slices brie cheese
- 2 tbsp freshly chopped mint leaves

Directions:

- Heat 1 tablespoon of olive oil in a medium skillet over medium heat until starting to smoke. Reduce the heat to low and sauté the onions until golden brown. Pour in the vinegar, maple syrup, and salt. Cook with frequent stirring to prevent burning until the onions caramelize, 20 minutes. Transfer to a plate and set aside.

- Heat the remaining olive oil in the same skillet, season the mushroom with salt and black pepper, and cook in the oil until cooked and brown on the outside, 10 to 12 minutes.

- Put a brie slice on each meat and top with the caramelized onions. Allow the cheese to melt for 2 to 3 minutes.

- Carefully spoon the meat with topping onto serving plates and garnish with the mint leaves.

- Serve immediately with buttered radishes.

Nutrition:

Calories:680 | Total Fat:71.8g | Saturated Fat:20.9g | Total Carbs:10g | Dietary Fiber:7g | Sugar:2g | Protein:3g | Sodium:525mg

Brown Rice Stir Fry with Vegetables

Preparation Time: 10-75 minutes | Cooking Time: 25 minutes | Servings: 4

Ingredients:

- 1 handful fresh parsley, chopped
- 1/2 zucchini, chopped
- 2 tablespoons olive oil
- 2 tablespoons soy sauce
- 1/2 bell pepper, chopped
- 1/2 cup brown rice, uncooked
- 4 garlic cloves, minced
- 1 cup red cabbage, chopped
- 1/8 teaspoon cayenne powder
- 1/2 broccoli head, chopped
- Sesame seeds, for garnish

Directions:

- Cook the brown rice as per the package instructions.

- Bring water to a boil in a frying pan and then add veggies and make sure they are fully covered with water. Cook for 1-2 minutes on high heat, and then drain the water and set aside.

- Add oil to the wok pan and heat over high heat and then add garlic along with parsley and cayenne powder. Cook for a minute stirring frequently and then add the drained veggies, tamari, and the cooked rice.

- Cook for 1-2 minutes and then garnish with sesame seeds if desired. Serve and enjoy!

Nutrition:

Calories: 140 Cal | Fat: 0.9 g | Carbs: 27.1 g | Protein: 6.3 g | Fiber: 6.2 g

Grilled Veggie Skewers

Preparation Time: 10-75 minutes | Cooking Time: 15 minutes | Servings: 4-6

Ingredients:

- 1 red onion, peeled, chopped
- 2 tablespoons avocado oil
- 2 portobello mushrooms, chopped
- 1 sweet potato, chopped
- 2 bell peppers, chopped
- 6 baby red potatoes, quartered
- Salt and black pepper, to taste
- 4 ears corn

Directions:

- Preheat the oven to 375F and add the sweet potato to a cooking pot along with the quartered potatoes and water. Bring to a boil and cook until lightly tender for about 10 minutes. When done, drain the water and let cool a bit.

- Thread the vegetables onto skewers, and then brush them evenly with oil. When done, season the vegetables generously with salt and pepper on each side.

- Cook the vegetables for about 10-15 minutes until tender and cooked through. Flip halfway. Place the corn directly on the vegetables to cook together.

- When done, serve and enjoy with the desired sauce.

Nutrition:

Calories:680 | Total Fat:71.8g | Saturated Fat:20.9g | Total Carbs:10g | Dietary Fiber:7g | Sugar:2g | Protein:3g | Sodium:525mg

Eggplant Teriyaki Bowls

Preparation Time: 10-75 minutes | Cooking Time: 45 minutes | Servings: 4

Ingredients:

- 1 carrot, shredded
- 1 chunky eggplant
- ¼ cup edamame beans, frozen
- 1 lime, ½ sliced, ½ juiced
- 2 spring onions, chopped
- 1 ½ tablespoon vegetable oil
- 1 handful radishes, sliced
- 1 tablespoon caster sugar
- 1 garlic clove, crushed
- ½ cup jasmine rice
- 2 tablespoons sesame seeds, toasted
- 1 small ginger, grated
- 2 tablespoons soy sauce

Directions:

- Add 2 cups of water to a cooking pan, add rice and salt to taste. Bring to a boil, cook for a minute, and then close the lid. Reduce the heat to low and cook for 10 minutes until cooked through. Turn off the heat and steam for an additional 10 minutes.

- Add a tablespoon of oil to a bowl and toss the eggplant in it. Preheat the wok pan, add the eggplant, and cook for 5 minutes, stirring often, until slightly softened and charred. Add the carrots to the wok along with garlic, ginger, and spring onions, and then fry for 2-3 minutes.

- In a small bowl, whisk the sugar along with soy sauce and a cup of water, and then add it into the wok. Simmer until the eggplant is very soft, for about 10-15 minutes.

- Add water to the pan and bring to a boil and then add the frozen edamame beans, remove the beans, drain and rinse them well under running water. Add the radishes to a bowl, drain the beans again, and then add them to the radishes. Squeeze lime juice on top and toss well until combined.

- Serve the rice in the bowls and then scoop the eggplant and sauce on top along with the beans and radishes. Sprinkle with sesame seeds and garnish with the lime slices. Enjoy

Nutrition:
Calories: 140 Cal | Fat: 0.9 g | Carbs: 27.1 g | Protein: 6.3 g | Fiber: 6.2 g

Quinoa and Black Bean Chilli

Preparation Time: 10-75 minutes | Cooking Time: 45 minutes | Servings: 8

Ingredients:

- 3 cups vegetable stock
- 1 onion, chopped
- 1 cup quinoa, rinsed, drained
- 1 red chili, chopped
- 2 teaspoons ground cumin
- 1 lb. tomatoes, chopped
- olive oil spray
- 1 teaspoon smoked paprika
- 1 small avocado, sliced
- ½ teaspoon chili powder
- 2 garlic cloves, crushed
- 1 lb. black beans, rinsed, drained
- Coriander leaves, to serve

Directions:

- Generously grease the cooking pan with oil and place over medium heat and then add the onion, red chili, and garlic. Fry the ingredients until soft, and then add spices and stir.

- Add the vegetable stock into the pan along with quinoa, black beans, and tomatoes, and then adjust the seasonings if needed.

- Close the lid and simmer until quinoa is tender, for about 30 minutes.

- When done, garnish with coriander leaves and top with the avocado slices. Serve and enjoy!

Nutrition:

Calories: 140 Cal | Fat: 0.9 g | Carbs: 27.1 g | Protein: 6.3 g | Fiber: 6.2 g

Broccoli Mac and Cheese

Preparation Time: 10-75 minutes | Cooking Time: 20 minutes | Servings: 4

Ingredients:

- 8 oz. whole-grain macaroni elbows, cooked
- 1 head of broccoli, florets
- 1 ½ tablespoon avocado oil
- 1 onion, chopped
- 1 cup potato, peeled and grated
- 3 cloves garlic, minced
- ½ teaspoon garlic powder
- ½ teaspoon onion powder
- ½ teaspoon dry mustard powder
- 1 small pinch of red pepper flakes
- ⅔ cup raw cashews
- 1 cup water, or more if needed
- ¼ cup nutritional yeast
- 3 teaspoons apple cider vinegar

- salt

Directions:

- Place a large pot over medium heat. Add salt and water and bring to a boil.

- Add broccoli and cook for 5 minutes. Once done, drain excess liquid and set aside in a large mixing bowl.

- Place a large skillet over medium heat. Add oil.

- Add onion, salt and cook for about 5 minutes.

- Add potatoes, garlic, garlic powder, onion powder, mustard powder, salt, red pepper flakes and cook for 60 seconds.

- Add cashews, water, bring the mixture to a simmer, reduce the heat, and let it cook until potatoes are tender. Remove from the heat.

- Pour the mixture into a food processor, add nutritional yeast, vinegar, and pulse until the mixture is smooth, adding water if necessary.

- Serve cooked pasta in bowls, topped with the blended mixture.

Nutrition:

Calories:680 | Total Fat:71.8g | Saturated Fat:20.9g | Total Carbs:10g | Dietary Fiber:7g | Sugar:2g | Protein:3g | Sodium:525mg

Butternut Squash Linguine with Fried Sage

Preparation Time: 10-75 minutes | Cooking Time: 25 minutes | Servings: 4

Ingredients:

- 3 cups butternut squash, peeled, seeded, and chopped
- 2 cups vegetable broth
- 12 oz. whole-grain fettuccine, cooked, 1 cup cooking liquid saved
- 1 onion, chopped
- 2 garlic cloves, pressed
- 2 tablespoons olive oil
- 1 tablespoon fresh sage, chopped
- 1/8 teaspoon red pepper flakes
- salt and pepper

Directions:

- Place a large pan over medium heat. Add oil.

- Add sage and cook it until crispy. Season with salt and set aside.

- Return the same pan to medium heat, add butternut, onion, garlic, red pepper flakes, salt, and pepper. Cook for about 10 minutes.

- Add broth and bring to a boil, then reduce the heat and let it cook for 20 minutes. • Place a pot of salty water over medium heat.

- Cool the squash mixture and blend the mixture until smooth with a mixer.

- Add pasta, ¼ cup reserved pasta liquid to the pan, return pan to medium heat and cook for 3 minutes.

Nutrition:

Calories: 140 Cal | Fat: 0.9 g | Carbs: 27.1 g | Protein: 6.3 g | Fiber: 6.2 g

Paella

Preparation Time: 10-75 minutes | Cooking Time: 1 hour | Servings: 6

Ingredients:

- 15 oz. diced tomatoes, drained
- 2 cups short-grain brown rice
- 1 ½ cups cooked chickpeas
- 3 cups vegetable broth
- ⅓ cup dry white wine
- 1 14 oz. artichokes, drained and chopped
- ½ cup Kalamata olives pitted and halved
- ¼ cup parsley, chopped
- ½ cup peas
- 3 tablespoons extra-virgin olive oil, divided
- 1 onion, chopped
- 6 garlic cloves, pressed or minced
- 2 teaspoons smoked paprika

- ½ teaspoon saffron threads, crumbled

- 2 bell peppers, stemmed, seeded, and sliced

- 2 tablespoons lemon juice

- salt and pepper

Directions:

- Preheat the oven to 350F.

- Place a large skillet over medium heat and add 2 tablespoons of oil.

- Add onion, salt and cook for 5 minutes.

- Add garlic, paprika and cook for ½ a minute.

- Add tomatoes and stir well. Cook until the mixture starts to thicken.

- Add rice and cook for 1 minute while stirring.

- Add chickpeas, broth, wine, saffron, and salt to taste. Increase the heat and bring the mixture to a boil. Remove from the heat.

- Cover and immediately transfer to an oven on the lower rack. Bake for 1 hour.

- Prepare a baking sheet by lining it with parchment paper. Combine artichokes, peppers, olives, 1 tablespoon olive oil, salt, and pepper. Mix well and roast vegetables on the upper rack in the oven for 45 minutes.

• Add parsley and lemon juice to the baking pan and mix well.

• Sprinkle the roasted vegetables and peas on the baked rice.

Nutrition:

Calories: 140 Cal | Fat: 0.9 g | Carbs: 27.1 g | Protein: 6.3 g | Fiber: 6.2 g

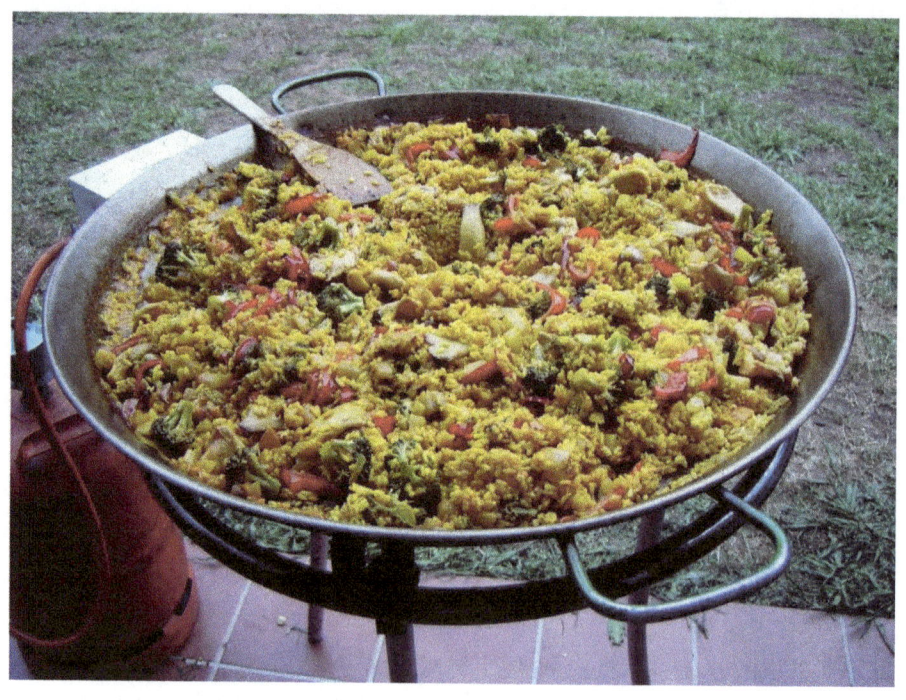

Spicy Thai Peanut Sauce Over Roasted Sweet Potatoes and Rice

Preparation Time: 10-75 minutes | Cooking Time: 1 hour 30 minutes | Servings: 4

Ingredients:

For the spicy Thai peanut sauce:

- ½ cup creamy peanut butter

- ¼ cup reduced-sodium tamari

- 3 tablespoons apple cider vinegar

- 2 tablespoons honey or maple syrup

- 1 teaspoon grated fresh ginger

- 2 cloves garlic, pressed

- ¼ teaspoon red pepper flakes

- 2 tablespoons water

For the roasted vegetables:

- 2 sweet potatoes, peeled and sliced

- 1 bell pepper, cored, deseeded, and sliced

- about 2 tablespoons coconut oil (or olive oil)
- ¼ teaspoon cumin powder
- salt

For the rice and garnishes:

- 1 ¼ cup jasmine brown rice
- 2 green onions, sliced
- a handful of cilantro, torn
- a handful of peanuts, crushed

Directions:

- Place a pot of water on medium heat and bring it to a boil.
- Preheat the oven to 425F.
- On a rimmed baking sheet, mix sweet potato, 1 tablespoon coconut oil, cumin, and salt. Roast in the middle rack for about 35 minutes.
- On another baking sheet, mix bell pepper with 1 teaspoon coconut oil, salt and mix well. Roast on the top rack for about 20 minutes until tender.
- When water is boiling in the pot add rice and mix well. Cook for about 30 minutes and drain excess liquid. Once done, cover and let it sit for 10 minutes, fluff it after.

- Mix sauce ingredients in a small bowl and set aside.

- Divide rice, roasted vegetables in bowls and top with sauce, green onions, cilantro, and peanuts before serving.

Nutrition:

Calories:680 | Total Fat:71.8g | Saturated Fat:20.9g | Total Carbs:10g | Dietary Fiber:7g | Sugar:2g | Protein:3g | Sodium:525mg

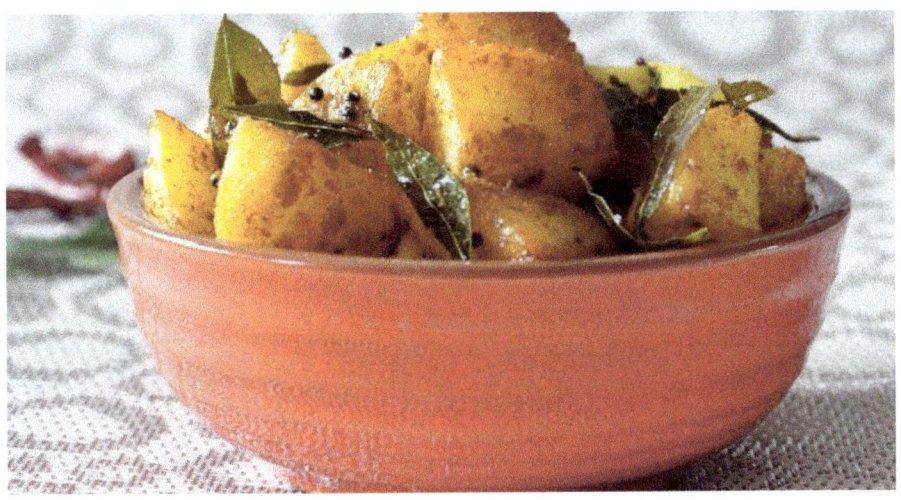

Chickpea Biryani

Preparation Time: 10-75 minutes | Cooking Time: 40 minutes | Servings: 6

Ingredients:

- 4 cups veggie stock
- 2 cups basmati rice, rinsed
- 1 can chickpeas, drained, rinsed
- ½ cup raisins
- 1 large onion, thinly sliced
- 2 cups thinly sliced veggies (bell pepper, zucchini, and carrots)
- 3 garlic cloves, chopped
- 1 tablespoon ginger, chopped
- 1 tablespoon cumin
- 1 tablespoon coriander
- 1 teaspoon chili powder
- 1 teaspoon cinnamon
- ½ teaspoon cardamom

- ½ teaspoon turmeric
- 2 tablespoons olive oil
- 1 bay leaf
- salt

Directions:

- Place a large skillet over medium-high heat. Add oil.
- Sauté onions for about 5 minutes.
- Reduce the heat to medium, add vegetables, garlic, and ginger. Cook for 5 minutes. Scoop 1 cup of this mixture and set aside.
- Add spices, bay leaf, and rice. Stir for about 1 minute.
- Add stock and salt to taste.
- Add chickpeas, raisins, and 1 cup of vegetables. Bring the mixture to a simmer over high heat.
- Lower the heat, cover tightly, and let it simmer for ½ an hour. Remove from the heat when rice is done.

Nutrition:

Calories: 140 Cal | Fat: 0.9 g | Carbs: 27.1 g | Protein: 6.3 g | Fiber: 6.2 g

Chinese Eggplant

Preparation Time: 10-75 minutes | Cooking Time: 45 minutes | Servings: 4

Ingredients:
- 1 ½ lbs. eggplants, chopped
- 2 cups of water
- 2 tablespoons cornstarch
- 4 tablespoons peanut oil
- 4 cloves garlic, chopped
- 2 teaspoons ginger, minced
- 10 dried red chilies
- salt
- For the Szechuan sauce:
- 1 teaspoon Szechuan peppercorns
- ¼ cup of soy sauce
- 1 tablespoon garlic chili paste
- 1 tablespoon sesame oil
- 1 tablespoon rice vinegar
- 1 tablespoon Chinese cooking wine
- 3 tablespoons coconut sugar
- ½ teaspoon five-spice

Directions:

- Place chopped eggplants in a shallow bowl. Add water and 2 teaspoons of salt. Stir cover and let it sit for about 15 minutes.

- Meanwhile, place a small pan over medium heat. Toast the Szechuan peppercorns for about 2 minutes and crush them.

- Add crushed peppercorns to a medium bowl, add soy, chili paste, sesame oil, rice vinegar, Chinese cooking vinegar, coconut sugar, and five spices.

- Drain excess liquid from the eggplants and toss in the corn starch.

- Place a large skillet over medium heat, add eggplants and cook them until golden. Set aside.

- Add 1 tablespoon of oil to the skillet placed over medium heat. Cook garlic and ginger for 2 minutes.

- Add dried chilies and cook for 1 minute. Add the Szechuan sauce and bring the mixture to a simmer in 20 seconds.

- Add back eggplants and cook for about 60 seconds.

Nutrition:

Calories:680 | Total Fat:71.8g | Saturated Fat:20.9g | Total Carbs:10g | Dietary Fiber:7g | Sugar:2g | Protein:3g | Sodium:525mg

Black Pepper Tofu with Bok Choy

Preparation Time: 10-75 minutes | Cooking Time: 30 minutes | Servings: 2

Ingredients:

- 12 oz. firm tofu, cubed
- 1/3 cup cornstarch for dredging
- 2 tablespoons coconut oil
- 1 teaspoon freshly cracked peppercorns
- 1 shallot, sliced
- 4 cloves garlic, chopped
- 6 oz. baby bok choy, sliced into 4 slices
- For the black pepper sauce:
- 2 tablespoons soy sauce
- 2 tablespoons Chinese cooking wine
- 2 tablespoons water
- 1 teaspoon brown sugar

- ½ teaspoon freshly cracked peppercorns
- 1 teaspoon chili paste

Directions:

- In a small bowl, combine wok sauce ingredients and mix well until sugar dissolves. Set aside.

- Place cornstarch in a shallow bowl and dredge tofu in the cornstarch. Set aside.

- Place a large skillet over medium heat. Heat 1 tablespoon coconut oil.

- Add peppercorns and toast for about 1 minute.

- Add tofu and cook on all sides for about 6 minutes. Set tofu aside.

- Add the remaining coconut oil. Add shallots, garlic, and bok choy. Cook for 8 minutes. • Add back the tofu and cook for less than a minute.

Nutrition:

Calories: 140 Cal | Fat: 0.9 g | Carbs: 27.1 g | Protein: 6.3 g | Fiber: 6.2 g

Lightning Source UK Ltd.
Milton Keynes UK
UKHW020644010621
384724UK00004B/42